Coconut Oil: A Guide to Healthy Fat and the Healing Power of Coconut Oil

What You Need To Know About Coconut Oil

I0449793

By: Marcia G. Dawkins

9781631871634

PUBLISHERS NOTES

Disclaimer – Speedy Publishing LLC

Speedy Publishing LLC

40 E Main Street,

Newark

Delaware

19711

Contact Us: 1-888-248-4521

Website: http://www.speedypublishing.co

REPRINTED Paperback Edition: ISBN: 9781631871634

Manufactured in the United States of America

DEDICATION

This book is dedicated to my friends and family members who were very supportive of me during my research on the properties and benefits of Coconut Oil. This book is also dedicated to persons seeking to lead a healthier lifestyle, through the use of natural products. It is hoped that the information provided in this book will be as enlightening and beneficial to you as it has been to me.

CONTENTS

INTRODUCTION - EXPLORING THE HEALTH BENEFITS OF COCONUT OIL

The coconut tree is one of the most versatile plants in existence. Whilst we are all familiar with the coconut as a food source, not many of us know the myriad of other benefits the coconut holds. In many countries coconut husks are woven into fabrics for mats, insulation and much more. The shells themselves are used as bowls, to make utensils and as floatation devices for rafts. Yet it is the coconut itself that draws the most interest. Coconut flesh has a beautiful taste and is used all over the world in a variety of cooking styles. Coconut milk is gorgeous to drink on its own and also is the chief ingredient in curries all over the world.

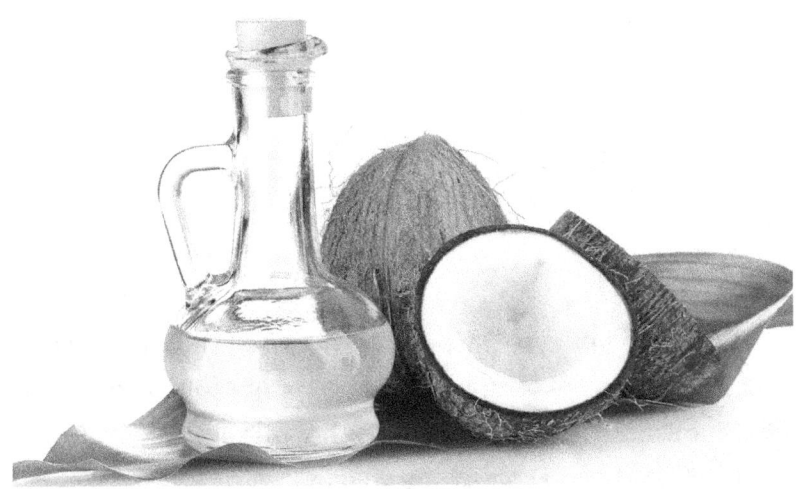

Over the years there have been many, many claims made about the natural health benefits of coconut oil mostly surrounding the dietary and medicinal properties that it holds. This is why in the west coconut oil has quickly become a hot consumer product with thousands of companies including it in their beauty products and thousands of recipes including it as an alternative to other oils.

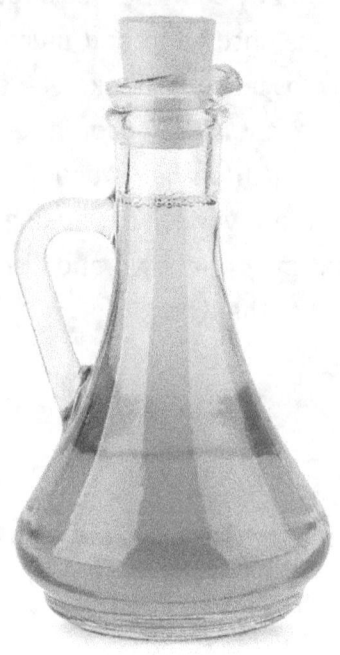

Yet a lot of controversy still surrounds the actual health benefits of coconut and debates still exist as to whether claims of its benefits have been exaggerated. This is where this book comes into play. We have carefully researched the benefits of coconut oil and outlined at length all the fantastic qualities that can come from eating coconut oil and applying it to your skin. We have left out some purported benefits through lack of evidence to support them and hope that this book will go some way to dispelling the myths surrounding coconut oil, whilst providing the reader with knowledge of coconut oil treatments that will be applicable to everyone in their normal lives.

Thank you for purchasing this book and we hope it will help you as it has helped us.

CHAPTER 1- COCONUT OIL: THE KEY TO IMPROVED IMMUNE HEALTH

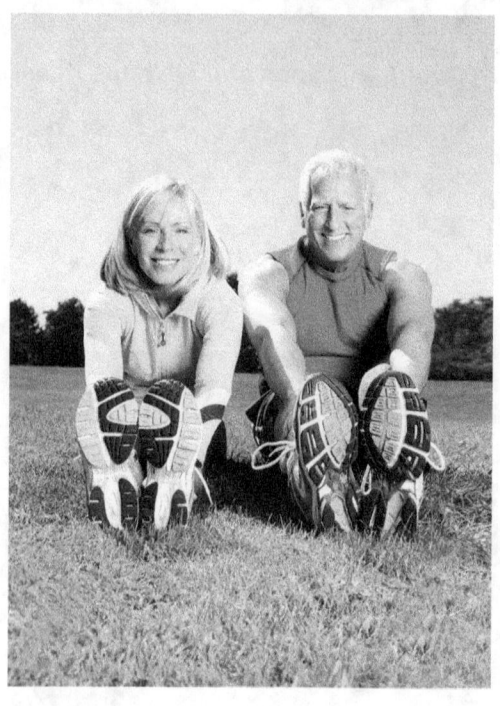

Maintaining a well-balanced diet and carefully monitoring your daily food and drink intake are central to keeping a well-balanced and healthy immune system. Your immune system has to fight off scores of bacteria every day and having a low immune system means you are more likely to catch viruses and other illnesses.

Ingesting coconut oil can help your immune system in a surprising number of ways.

Coconut oil has great natural health benefits and works as an effective cure for a number of common illnesses including eczema, indigestion and a variety of skin diseases like age spot. However coconut oil can also aid your immune system in a number of surprising ways.

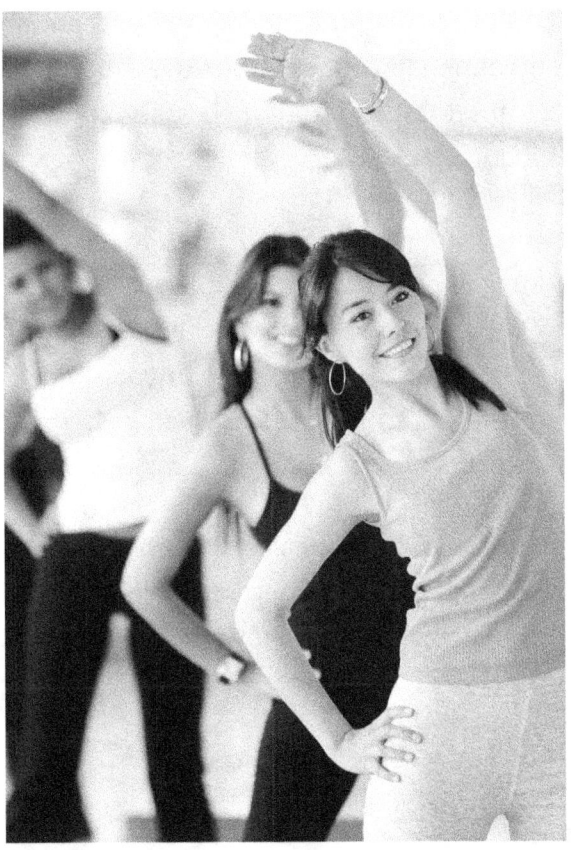

The key way coconut oil can boost your immune system is through the ingestion of saturated fats- the most beneficial of which are - medium chain triglycerides. These are the most easily digestible saturated fats as the body transports them straight to the liver where they are not used for the production of fat, so you don't have to be overly worried about increasing your cholesterol as you boost your immune system.

Medium chain triglycerides are used by your immune system to create antimicrobials - which we more commonly think of as antibodies. Antibodies are the primary defense mechanism your body has when fighting infections and viruses so having moderate amounts of saturated fats is necessary to keep your antibody production up.

The fats in coconut oil contain antimicrobial lipids which have anti-viral and anti-fungal properties. Coconut oil contains Lauric, Caprylic and Capric acids which, when broken down, are converted into specific antibodies used to in your body's defenses against a range of diseases including herpes, influenza and other infections/diseases.

Having the right antibodies to fight specific bacteria is central to your body's wellbeing so adding some coconut oil to your diet is an easy way to ensure you stay happy and healthy.

CHAPTER 2- THE BEST ALTERNATIVE FOR A HEALTHY HEART

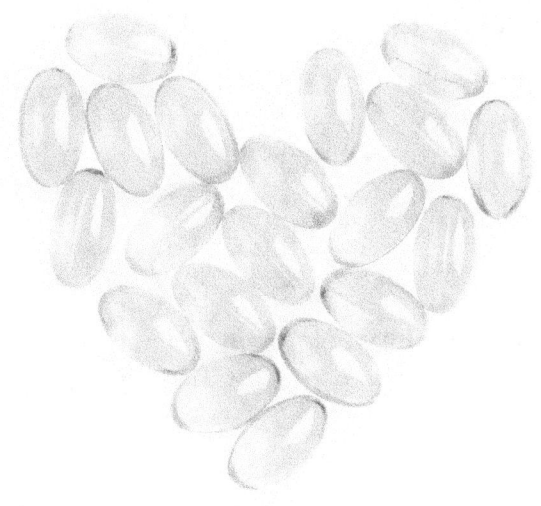

In this last section we're going to be examining the claimed benefits of coconut oil in relation to the prevention of heart disease. This is perhaps the most widely contested area of debate in coconut oil research. The high amount of saturated fats in coconut oil would seem to indicate that it would have a negative impact on your health by creating more fatty tissues. However research into the chemical composition of these saturated fats has shown that they are primarily medium chain triglycerides, the least harmful, and most beneficial, form of saturated fats your body can use.

Worldwide cardiovascular disease causes over 12.5 million deaths a year whilst in the US over 60 million people suffer some form of cardiovascular (heart) disease. The most common form of this disease is coronary artery disease which results from the build-up of fat, plaque and scar tissue around the arteries. The most common causes of cardiovascular disease are;

- High cholesterol
- Heredity
- Smoking
- Obesity
- High blood pressure
- Diabetes

This means that coconut oil would seem an unlikely candidate as a dietary supplement to decrease your risk of heart disease but it actually isn't.

This is all do with the type of saturated fats we ingest on a regular basis. Sri Lankans for example have the lowest risk of cardiovascular disease in the world and their primary cooking oil comes from coconuts. This may seem incidental but there has been a marked increase in cardiovascular disease in Sri Lanka and India that fits with the increased use of vegetable oils which have replaced traditional cooking aids and consumables.

The saturated fats in most western diets are of a far worse kind. These are high chain triglycerides that the body cannot break down as efficiently as medium chains. This means that they build up as fatty deposits around your heart and arteries increasing the risk of coronary heart disease. Replacing your oils and margarines with coconut oil therefore actually decreases your risk of heart disease and will help you lose weight.

Clearly then we can see that despite appearance coconut oil is actually a better alternative to other oils and should definitely be used as often as possible in order to improve your diet and reduce the risks of heart diseases.

Chapter 3- Coconut Oil: The Key to Improved Digestion

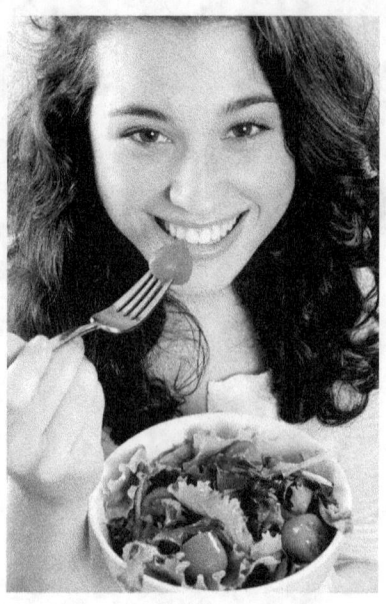

Coconut oil has long been held to be a useful supplement to aid in digestion. This is one of the key reasons it is the primary ingredient in many curry sources – and why curry goes down so well.

As we have seen in previous chapters coconut oil has strong anti-microbial benefits which when ingested help you to fight off nasty bacteria and bolster your immune system.

Many digestive problems are caused by the presence of microbes in the food we eat. We have a natural set of microbes in our stomach acid that aid digestion but these often react negatively with certain enzymes found in other foods.

This means that the key way virgin coconut oil can help our digestion is by curing indigestion.

Indigestion is primarily caused by acid in your stomach irritating the stomach lining and the top of your small intestine. The most common process that causes it is known as acid reflux. This is most commonly caused by bad diet and obesity as well as stomach ulcers and other stomach infections.

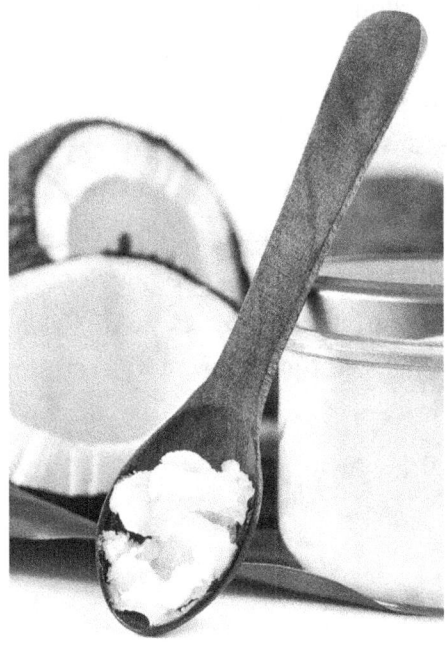

The saturated fats in coconut oil, especially Lauric acid and Capric acid, aid your stomach, and digestive track, in neutralizing micro bacteria. These fats help remove parasitic bacteria and fungi keeping your digestive tract and stomach at its optimal performance.

Coconut Oil

Whilst these benefits are great if you have indigestion they also help the clean and healthy running of the rest of your body too. Coconut oil is rich in vitamins and minerals itself but the fatty acids within it actually encourage the absorption of most other vitamins and minerals into your body. This is because the enzymes that are released when the fatty acid chains break down act as a catalyst for the absorption of other vitamins and minerals.

But before you go guzzling gallons of coconut oil be aware that this would have a negative impact on your overall health. Whilst coconut oil is a great way to cure indigestion and is beneficial to your digestive system in general, over-use of coconut oil can have negative consequences. This is because whilst the saturated fats in virgin coconut oil are not unhealthy in small doses large amounts will be equivalent to eating lots of unhealthy meat and dairy products. So it is best to use coconut oil in cooking without pouring the entire bottle over every meal.

Chapter 4- Coconut Oil: The Natural Metabolism Booster.

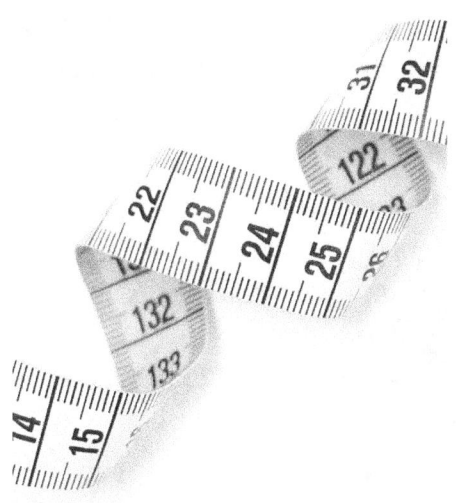

Many people think that because virgin coconut oil has a high proportion of saturated fat it is bad for you to eat.

This is one of the greatest myths surrounding coconut oil and now turn to dispelling this myth and seeing how you can use coconut oil as a an aid to weight loss.

The chemical make-up of coconut fats

90% of coconut oil is saturated fat. Sounds like a nightmare, doesn't it, but a closer examination reveals the surprising truth.

Coconut Oil

This is because most of the saturated fatty acids in coconut oil are what are known as medium chain triglycerides. Medium chain triglycerides are actually easier for your body to break down than other saturated fats. Especially those found in fast food and other artificially created products. This is because there are fundamental differences in the chain composition in these fats which mean they are harder for your body to breakdown - which in turn means they are more likely to accumulate in your arteries and in your skin tissue.

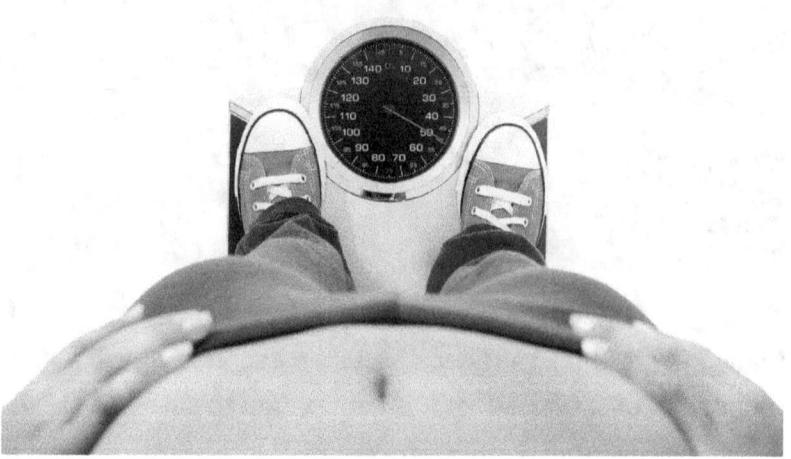

Further, the saturated fats in coconut oil - especially the Lauric acid actually increase the body's metabolism and promote optimal health of the thyroid and enzymes systems. Having a high metabolism means that the body burns calories at an increased rate. This is due to the acidity of your stomach acid and how effectively it can convert food to energy. Having a healthy gut will greatly increase your chances of having a high metabolism and help you start shedding weight.

The enzymes contained within coconut oil actually act as catalysts to your stomach acid and help you break down fat at an increased rate- and as your metabolism is also increased you can burn a higher proportion of the calories you take in. They also help to promote a healthy gut by fighting bacteria and strengthening the stomach lining. Hence coconut oil actually is much better for you to use in cooking and food than other alternatives as it has added benefits not found in vegetable and olive oil.

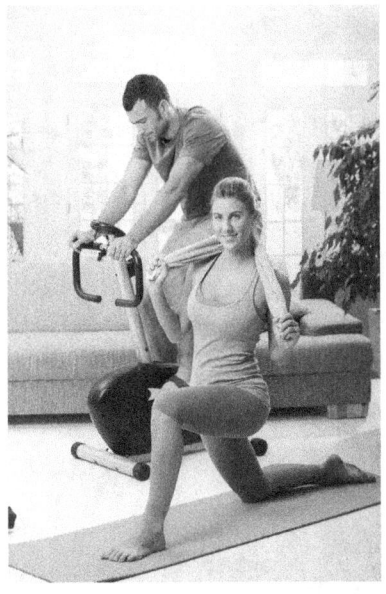

Virgin coconut oil as it contains 50% Lauric acid is definitely well worth including in your diet. The easiest ways to do this are to replace your cooking oil with coconut oil - which incidentally is much more complimentary to the tastes of many foods, especially curries and stir-fries. Alternatively you

Coconut Oil

can also use coconut milk more regularly in your cooking as it can be a key ingredient in a variety of delicious curries.

CHAPTER 5- TREATING INFECTIONS WITH COCONUT OIL

We've already seen that coconut oil can help fight a variety of infections and that it aids your immune system thanks to the fatty acids such as lauric acid and capric acid. However the natural health benefits of coconut oil actually go far beyond this as it is a versatile treatment for a variety of internal and external infections. It is these we are going to examine in this chapter.

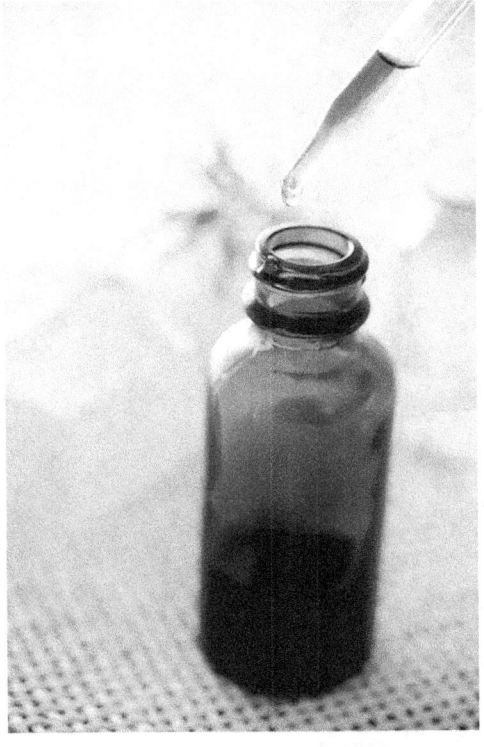

Firstly then externally coconut oil can be used to treat a variety of skin afflictions and is brilliant for cuts, scrapes and bruises.

Coconut Oil

On your skin virgin coconut oil is aptly suited to preventing common skin afflictions such as eczema and other rashes as it creates an impermeable layer of oil between your skin and the air. Whilst usually this would result in your skin becoming unhealthy and not being able to breathe properly the chemical composition of coconut oil actually aerates the skin and moisturizes it at the same time. You shouldn't keep yourself covered in coconut oil twenty four seven but applying a layer twice a day will keep your skin irritations safely at bay and leave you with healthier skin.

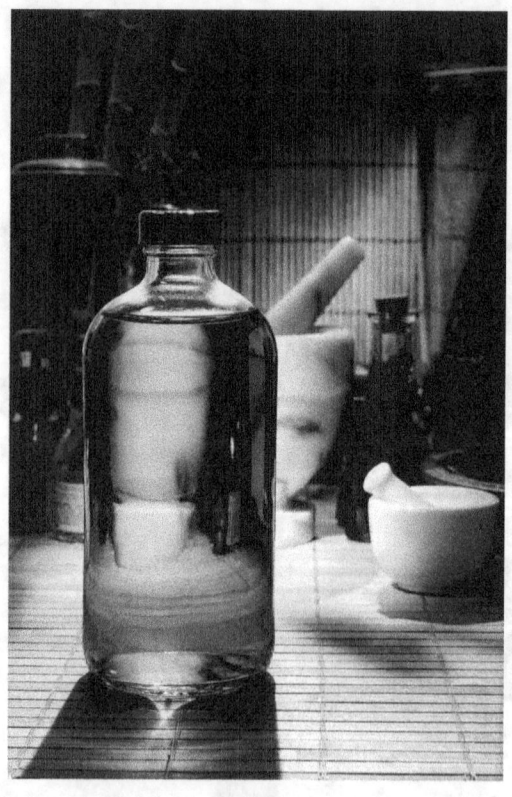

On cuts, bruises and scrapes virgin coconut oil helps in the same way as above - by keeping the area free from infection.

Yet the moisturizing effects also help heal the skin by giving it the nutrients it needs to rejuvenate and repair skin tissue. The nutrients in coconut oil not only help heal your skin but they also help tighten the skin - this is great for removing stretch marks and minimizing scar tissue.

Secondly the enzymes in coconut oil are known to kill many viruses including influenza, measles, herpes, hepatitis and SARS. This means that coconut oil can actually protect you from catching some of the worst diseases we are exposed to in the modern world. The enzymes work by simply decomposing the harmful bacteria- thereby neutralizing any potential they have to create negative effects.

Thirdly coconut oil is a great treatment for candidiasis and other yeast infections.

Organic coconut oil is one of the most efficient natural health aids in fighting candida off completely. Changing your diet in this simple way can really help relieve you of candiasis forever.

Candida is notoriously hard to remove from the body as the source of the infection is not necessarily the same as the location of the infection itself.

Candida grows in a low PH and overly toxic environment. If you are overweight, eat a lot of junk food or underweight and sedentary your bodies skin and immune system are less tolerant, meaning you are likely to develop candida or yeast infections much more frequently.

Coconut Oil

In your diet coconut oil helps bolster the immune system as well as being a much better source of saturated fat than junk food helping you to actually lose weight whilst still maintaining a balanced diet.

Applied externally the nutrients in coconut oil help to protect your skin and create a barrier to external free radicals meaning that repeat infections are unlikely. The topical application of coconut oil will also help soothe the skin meaning you won't suffer from as much irritation. Coconut oil acts as a fungicide by literally breaking down the fungus and stymying further fungal growth.

This makes coconut oil one of the best natural health remedies to a huge variety of common afflictions. It really is a wonder of the natural world and you'd be remiss not to buy some today.

Chapter 6- Coconut Oil: The Key to Healthier Hair

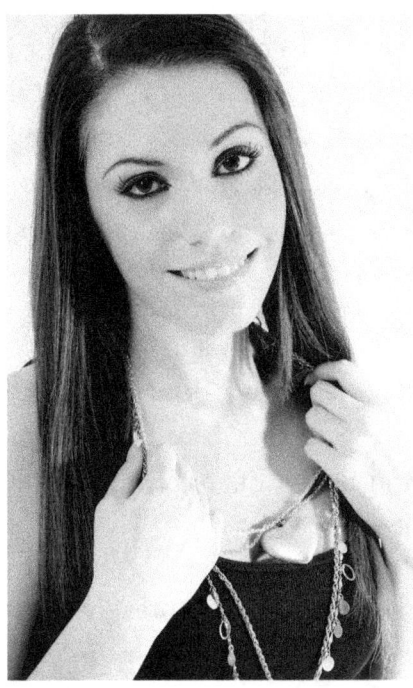

Coconut oil has long been regarded as one of the best hair conditioning natural health products in the natural world.

Many people worldwide use coconut oil as their sole hair conditioning product as it is relatively cheap and gives remarkable results.

The benefits of coconut oil for your hair are numerous. Coconut oil helps keep your hair fully moisturized; it promotes full growth and creates strong hair whilst keeping the scalp free from flakes. Its main benefit comes from increasing the protein retention in your hair – allowing for fuller and stronger growth.

Coconut Oil

Whilst many companies use tiny amounts of virgin coconut oil in their high end products a lot of people are now turning to pure virgin coconut oil for the benefits it brings.

The key benefits of using coconut oil or even coconut oil cream in your hair can be exposed by looking at the chemical properties of coconut oil. Often people proscribe coconut oil as a remedy for hair loss - or at least to slow the onset of hairless and we can soon see why.

Lauric acid

Lauric acid is found primarily in the oil produced from coconuts. One of the primary causes of hair loss and recession of the hair line is the action of microbes on the scalp and at the base of the follicles.

Lauric acid acts as an anti-microbial oil that prevents the build-up of damaging microbes thus preventing hair loss and stimulating fresh strong growth.

This means that not only is coconut oil great for your hair but it can also prevent the loss of hair if used regularly.

Capric acid

Virgin coconut oil contains a high yield of not only Lauric acid but Capric acid as well. Capric acid is another anti-microbe that works in a similar way to Lauric acid. It tackles microbes at the source preventing further spread and loss of hair whilst stimulating new hair growth.

Vitamin E

We all know how important vitamin E is to natural health generally. Vitamin E helps keep the skin in tip top condition and is one of the key ways in which your hair retains its shine and bounce.

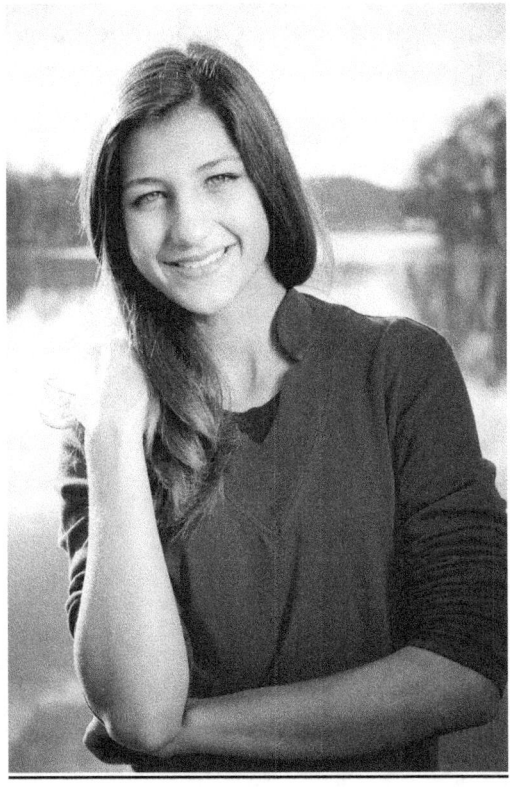

Fatty acids

The fatty acids in coconut oil serve as a great anti-dandruff mechanism that far outshines most anti-dandruff shampoos.

Coconut Oil

Regular application softens and moistens the skin reducing the accumulation of hair and flakes.

The benefits of virgin coconut oil for your hair are fantastic. This is why more and more people are replacing their traditional shampoos and conditioners with either pure or high density coconut oil products. Many people have now started using coconut oil for stylistic reasons as it acts in a similar way to hair wax or gel - without producing the flakes of typical wax and without damaging the hairs strength. This is due to coconut oils ability to retain moisture at almost all temperatures.

CHAPTER 7- COCONUT OIL: THE KEY TO YOUTHFUL SKIN

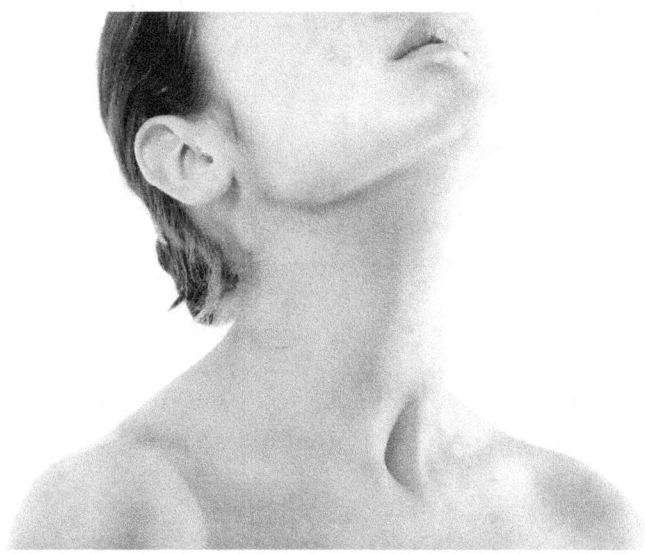

Coconut oils natural health benefits extend far beyond the fantastic benefits for your hair that we saw in the first section of this book.

Coconut oil has a large number of fantastic benefits for your skin as well.

The first as we have already seen is the great benefit of Vitamin E. Vitamin E keeps your skin healthy, spot free and protects against skin cancer.

Vitamin E in coconut oil acts as an antioxidant - meaning that it protects skin cells from UV light, pollution and the negative effects of smoke and other "free radicals". The most notable of these is of course the prevention of skin cancer making

Coconut Oil

coconut oil one of the most beneficial forms of sun screen available.

Vitamin E also helps reduce the appearance of stretch marks and prevents the appearance of age spots by rejuvenating the skin cells over your body.

As coconut oil has a high yield of vitamin E many people are now using it as a substantive replacement for expensive sun-creams, or as a supplement to sun screen as it is less harmful to the skin.

Coconut oil also has fantastic moisturizing benefits that extend beyond simply the high content of vitamin E.

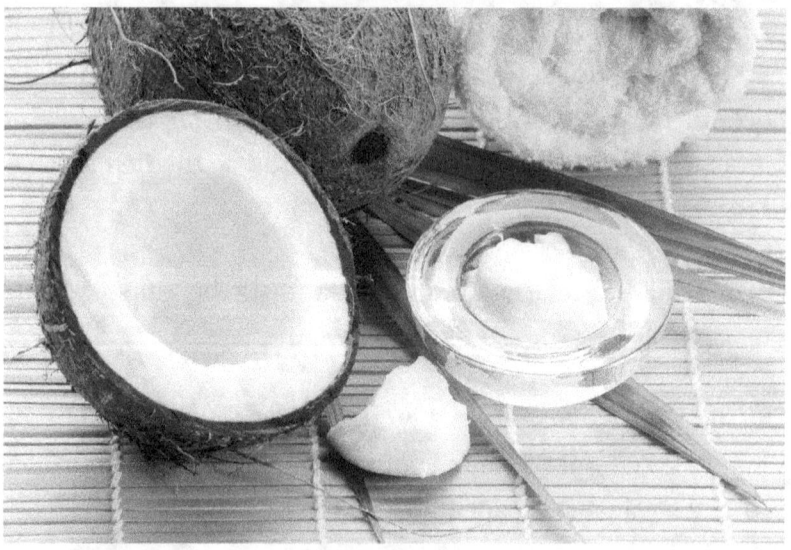

Virgin coconut oil is a highly effective and completely natural moisturizer. It is unlikely to create adverse reactions as it is completely natural meaning that, unlike many moisturizers, you don't have to worry about rashes and unsightly blemishes appearing on your skin. Further compared to most moisturizing creams - which let's face it carry extortionate price tag- coconut oil is cheap to buy and lasts a long time.

In terms of natural remedies coconut oil treats and alleviates many common skin conditions including eczema, dermatitis and psoriasis. This is why it is a common ingredient in skin treatments worldwide.

So by now you are probably thinking this is great I'll buy some, but there's actually more benefits to your skin from coconut oil still to come.

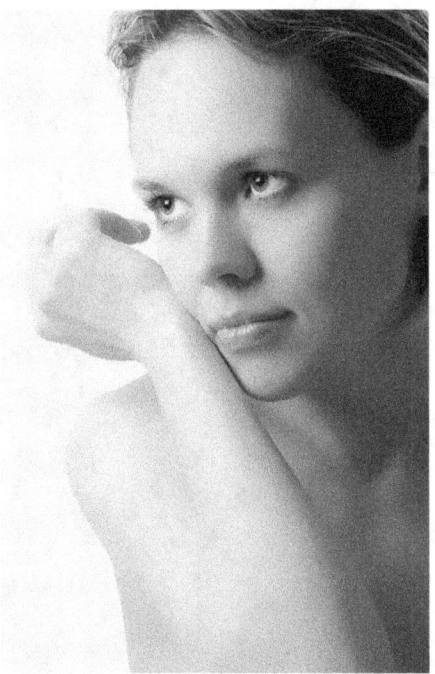

Finally then coconut oil actually works as an anti-ageing cream. The antioxidants of vitamin E provide an initial layer of

Coconut Oil

protection against the sun but the combination of this with the Lauric acid found in coconut oil keeps the skin bacteria free. This means that coconut oil is giving your skin a double helping of beneficial effects. This promotes anti-ageing skin as it fights off bacteria and strengthens the skin tissue.

Coconut oil really is a one of nature's most wonderful products.

ABOUT THE AUTHOR

Marcia G. Dawkins is an award-winning author, researcher, educator and speaker who has done extensive research on the properties of coconut oil and the benefits to be derived from its use.

In light of current debates and controversy surrounding the extent to which coconut oil significantly contributes to improved health, the author seeks to dispel the myths that are most commonly associated with coconut oil and its usage.

In this book, the author explores a number of ways in which coconut oil contributes to the reduction of certain health-related risk factors and the increase in overall health and wellbeing.

www.ingramcontent.com/pod-product-compliance
Lightning Source LLC
Chambersburg PA
CBHW061943280526
45787CB00004B/1703